Vega

How to Lose Weight Forever On a Vegan Diet for Beginners and Boost Immune System

(The Ultimate Vegan Recipe Book for Beginners)

Fred Ivey

Published by Robert Satterfield
Publishing House

© **Fred Ivey**

Vegan Diet: How to Lose Weight Forever On a Vegan Diet for Beginners and Boost Immune System (The Ultimate Vegan Recipe Book for Beginners)

ISBN 978-1-989682-91-3

Legal & Disclaimer

The information contained in this book is not designed to replace or take the place of any form of medicine or professional medical advice. The information in this book has been provided for educational and entertainment purposes only.

TABLE OF CONTENT

Part 1

Introduction

If you are tired of eating over-processed, over packaged foods and want to try a fresher, healthier, natural approach to eating vegan, then this cookbook is for you. Cooking vegan doesn't have to be difficult. The book offers easy to prepare and cook tasty vegan recipes that are loaded with vitamins, nutrients, and other beneficial micro-nutrients. Recent research shows that plant-based vegan diet is better for the health of the dieter and for the planet. The vegan diet comes with numerous health benefits and millions of dieters around the world have discovered the health benefits of the vegan diet.

As soon as you begin the diet, you will feel more vitalized, energetic and motivated. You will lose visible amount stubborn abdominal fat in weeks and lower your risk of various obesity-related diseases, including high blood pressure, heart disease, high cholesterol, type 2 diabetes and all types of cancer. Unlike other cookbooks, this book includes Nutrition Values with every recipe, so you can keep track of your healthy vegan lifestyle. This cookbook is not only for vegans, but also for the growing number of people who are looking to eat healthier, lighter and feeling full after each meal.

Chapter 1 How to Go Vegan

Becoming a vegan is not a simple dietary choice. Veganism is a philosophy and lifestyle choice. A vegan doesn't eat anything that is the animal origin and also avoid using any animal based products or clothes. Here are a few suggestions that will help you become a vegan.

Take your time: You have decided to become a vegan, so don't rush and go at your own pace. Some people can manage to go vegan right away; if this approach suits you, then it's great. However, don't worry if you can't make a quick transition to the vegan diet. Just like any other lifestyle change, going vegan takes getting used to and understanding which approach will be best for you also takes time. Making small changes is one of the easiest ways to incorporate vegan foods in your diet. For example, you can avoid meat and dairy one day a week and gradually progress from there. You can start by eating one vegan meal every day, then from the second week eat two vegan meal daily and so on.

- Take the right approach: While following the vegan diet, it is important that you don't miss out on important vitamins and essential nutrients. Just because you are eating vegan, doesn't mean you are eating healthy because there are a lot of vegan junk foods available. Plan your diet in such a way that you get every type of vitamins and nutrients your body needs.

- Experiment and try new things: Going vegan no way relates to less taste or flavor. Try new things and treat your taste buds to new foods and flavors. You don't have to become a skillful chef because vegan recipes are really simple and easy. Here are a couple of links for new dieters :for USA - Vegan Store, for UK Vegan Store.

- Don't hesitate and ask for help: Where to get vegan chocolate or how to bake cakes without eggs are some of the common questions new vegans ask.

You are not alone, so no worries. There are a lot of vegan Facebook and Twitter groups available. For any new vegan, this Website offers additional support for the first 30 days.

- Remember why you choose to become a vegan: It is important that you continue to remind yourself why you choose to become a vegan, even after a successful transition to a vegan diet. Often people find it relatively easy to transitioning to vegan. However, once they have a bad day, the whole vegan thing seems too much work. If you are having a bad day, then take deep breaths, relax and reflect on your choices and how much you have achieved so far. Watching informative videos on Veganism and reading books like this can be uplifting. Keeping photos of your favorite animals in your home and at your workplace also act as a motivation. Here is a video to keep you motivated on Veganism.

Vegan Basics

Vegans don't eat foods that come from animals, including dairy products and eggs. A vegan diet contains only plants such as vegetables, whole grains, nuts, fruits and other plant-based foods. Vegans are avoiding all animal-based products, so eating a balanced, healthy diet is important. Here is a guideline how you can eat a healthy vegan diet:

- Eat at least five portions of a variety of vegetables and fruits daily.
- Choose wholegrain where possible. Base meals on pasta, rice, bread, potatoes and other starchy carbohydrates.
- Eat some pulses, beans, and other proteins daily.
- Eat a few unsaturated spreads and oil.
- Have some dairy alternatives such as yogurts and soy drinks.
- Drink at least 8 glasses of water daily.

Getting the right nutrients when following the vegan diet

Plan your vegan diet properly, otherwise, you could miss out on essential nutrients, such as iron, calcium, omega-3 fatty acids and vitamin B12.

Vegan sources of omega- 3 fatty acids

Omega-3 fatty acids lower your risk of heart disease and make your heart healthy. Vegan sources of omega-3 are:

- Rapeseed oil
- Soya oil and soya-based foods
- Flaxseed
- Walnuts

Vegan sources of iron

Your body needs iron to produce enough red blood cells. Good sources of iron for vegans are:

- Whole-meal bread and flour
- Dark-green leafy vegetables such as spring greens, broccoli, and watercress.
- Dried fruits such as apricots, figs, and prunes
- Nut and pulses

Vegan sources of vitamin B12

Your body needs vitamin B12 to maintain a healthy nervous system and healthy blood flow throughout the body. Animal-based foods are the only natural source of vitamin B12. So you have to consume foods that are fortified with vitamin B12:

- Include vitamin B12 fortified cereals in your breakfast.
- A yeast extract – Marmite is fortified with vitamin B12
- Drink vitamin B12 fortified unsweetened soya drink.

Vegan sources of calcium

Your body needs calcium for healthy, stronger bones and teeth. As a vegan, you have to take calcium and vitamin D from non-animal sources, including:

- Calcium-set tofu
- Fortified, unsweetened soy, rice and oat drinks
- Sesame seeds and tahini
- Fortified bread products
- Dried fruits, such as raisins, prunes, apricots and figs
- Pulses

Vegan sources of vitamin D are

- Vitamin D supplements

- Vitamin D fortified unsweetened soya drinks, breakfast cereals, and fat spreads.
- 20 minutes of daily midday sun exposure will give your body enough natural vitamin D.

Shopping tips

- Check the labels of all packaged products such as stock cubes, spreads, sauces, and bouillon powder. Ingredients such as whey, casein and lactose are all derived from milk.
- Most bread and pastries contain butter and some contain milk.
- Non-vegan beer and wines can contain animal products.
- Replace gelatin with vege-gel or agar agar.

Chapter 2 Breakfast Recipes

Vegan Breakfast Burrito

Ingredients for 4 (3/4 cup) servings

- Extra-firm tofu – 1 package (rinsed, pressed and diced)
- Extra virgin olive oil – 1 teaspoon
- Garlic cloves – 3
- Diced sweet onion – 2 cups
- Diced potato – 1 cup
- Sliced Crimini mushrooms – 1.5 cups
- Nutritional yeast – ¼ cup
- Minced fresh basil – 3 to 4 tablespoons
- Minced fresh parsley – 2 tablespoons
- Fresh lemon juice – 1 to 1.5 tablespoons
- Kosher salt and black pepper to taste
- Green onion, salsa, chopped pineapple and Daiya cheese for garnish

Method
1. Heat 1 teaspoon oil in a large skillet over medium heat. Over medium heat, sauté onion and garlic for a few

minutes. Add in the mushrooms and potato and sauté for about 12 minutes. Stirring frequently and reducing heat if necessary.

2. Lower the heat to low and stir in lemon juice, tofu, yeast, fresh herbs and season with salt and pepper to taste. Continue to cook on low heat for a few more minutes, or until potato is cooked through.

3. Add ¾ cup of the tofu-mushroom mixture on a large tortilla wrap. Top with chopped green onion and cheese if desired.

Nutritional Information (¾ cup, with wrap and garnishes)
- Calories 182
- Fat 5g
- Carbs 22g
- Protein 17g

Chia Seed Breakfast Bowl

Ingredients for 2 servings

Chia mixture

- Chia seeds – 4 tablespoons
- Almond milk – 1 to 1.25 cups
- Small bananas – 2, chopped small
- Pure vanilla extract – ½ teaspoon
- Cinnamon – 2 pinches

Toppings

- Raw buckwheat groats – 2 tablespoons, soaked
- Raisins – 2 tablespoons, soaked
- Whole raw almonds – 2 tablespoons, chopped and soaked
- Cinnamon – 2 pinches
- Hemp seeds – 2 tablespoons

Method

1. Mash bananas in a bowl and stir in the chia seeds. Whisk in cinnamon, almond milk, and vanilla until combined. Cover and keep in the fridge overnight to thicken.

Into another bowl, add chopped almonds, raisins, and buckwheat groats. Cover with water and soak overnight on the counter or in the fridge.

2. In the morning, place chia pudding into a bowl. Add more almond milk if you want it thin or add more chia seeds to thicken it up.

3. Drain and rinse the almond/buckwheat mixture.
    Sprinkle on top of the chia mixture along with a tablespoon of hemp seeds and a pinch of cinnamon.

4. Drizzle with maple syrup and serve.

Nutritional Information Per Serving
- Calories 380
- Fat 19.2g
- Carbs 48.3g
- Protein 12.9g

Vegan Pancakes

Ingredients for 3 servings
- All-purpose flour – 1 ¼ cups
- White sugar – 2 tablespoons

- Baking powder – 2 teaspoons
- Salt – ½ teaspoon
- Water – 1 ¼ cups
- Oil – 1 tablespoon

Method
1. In a large bowl, stiff the flour, baking powder, sugar, and salt.

In a small bowl, whisk the oil and water together.

2. In the center of the dry ingredients, make a well and pour in the wet.
3. Stir until just blended. The mixture will be lumpy.

Lightly grease a griddle and heat over medium-high heat.

Add large spoonfuls of batter onto the griddle and cook until the edges are dry and bubbles form.

4. Flip and cook until browned on the other side.

Nutritional Information Per Serving
Calories 264
Fat 5.1g

Carbs 48.9g
Protein 5.4g

Vegan French Toast

Ingredients for 4 to 6 servings
- Vanilla-flavored soymilk – 1 cup
- Flour – 2 tablespoons
- Sugar – 1 tablespoon
- Nutritional yeast – 1 tablespoon
- Cinnamon – 1 teaspoon
- Bread – 4 to 6 slices (slightly stale)

Method
1. In a bowl, mix together the first 5 ingredients.

Dip a piece of bread in the mixture.
2. Coat well and cook on a skillet until golden-brown.
3. Repeat with the other slices.
4. Serve.

Nutritional Information Per Serving
- Calories 104.3
- Fat 1.1g

- Carbs 20.6g
- Protein 3.5g

Vegan Tortilla

Ingredients for 4 servings
- Extra virgin olive oil
- Medium potatoes – 28 oz. (sliced 1/8 inch thick)
- Onion – 1/2, diced
- Chickpea flour – 16 tablespoons
- Water – 16 tablespoons + 1 cup
- Salt to taste
- Dash of black salt

Method
1. Heat 1 or 2 tablespoons of olive oil in a non-stick frying pan.
Add the onion, potatoes, salt to taste and 1 cup of water and bring to boil.
2. Cook until potatoes are soft, about 20 minutes, stirring occasionally.
3. Remove the onion and potatoes from the pan.

In a bowl, add 16 tablespoons of water and 16 tablespoons of chickpea flour. Add the salt and beat with a fork.

Pour in onion/potato mixture. Mix well.

4. In a frying pan, add one or two tablespoons of olive oil and heat over medium heat.

5. Pour in the onion/potato mixture and cook over medium heat for 5 minutes.

Place a plate over the tortilla, then turn it around and cook the other side for 5 minutes more.

6. Turn the tortilla again if required.

7. Season with black salt and serve.

Nutritional Information Per Serving (1/4 of the recipe)

- Calories 310
- Fat 8.5g
- Carbs 49.9g
- Protein 9.4g

Mushroom, Spinach and Tofu Quiche

Ingredients for 8 servings

For the crust

- Ground flax – 1 tablespoon plus 3 tablespoons water (mixed together)
- Whole almonds – 1 cup, ground into flour
- Buckwheat groats or rolled oats – 1 cup, ground into flour
- Dried parsley – 1 teaspoon
- Dried oregano – 1 teaspoon
- Kosher salt – ½ teaspoon
- Olive oil – 1 tablespoon
- Water as needed

For the quiche

- Firm tofu – 1 block (14 oz.) rinsed and pressed
- Olive oil – 1 tablespoon
- Yellow onion or leek – 1, thinly sliced
- Garlic cloves – 3 large, minced

- Sliced Cremini mushrooms – 3 cups (8 oz.)
- Fresh chives – ½ cups, finely chopped
- Fresh basil leaves – ½ cup, finely chopped
- Oil-packed-sun-dried tomatoes – 1/3 cup, finely chopped
- Baby spinach - 1 cup
- Nutritional yeast – 2 tablespoons
- Dried oregano – 1 teaspoon
- Fine grain sea salt - ¾ to 1 teaspoon
- Black pepper to taste
- Red pepper flakes to taste

Method

1. Preheat the oven to 375F. Lightly grease a round 10-inch tart pan.
2. To make the crust: in a small bowl, whisk together flax and water and set aside.
3. In a large bowl, stir together the buckwheat flour, almond meal, oregano, parsley, and salt.
4. Add in the oil and flax mixture. Stir until mostly combined. Continue to add

water until it gets the consistency of a cookie dough.

5. Crumble the dough with your hands over the base of the tart pan. Starting from the center, press the mixture evenly into the pan. Poke several holes so the air can escape.

6. Bake in the preheated oven at 350F until lightly golden and firm to touch, about 13 to 16 minutes. Set aside to cool. Increase the oven temperature to 375F.

7. To make the filling: break apart the tofu block into 4 pieces, then add into a food processor. Process until smooth and creamy. Add some almond milk if necessary.

8. Add oil in a skillet and sauté the onion and garlic over medium heat for a few minutes.

9. Stir in the mushrooms and season with salt. Cook for 10 to 12 minutes, or until most of the water cooks off the mushrooms.

10. Stir in the sun-dried tomatoes, herbs, oregano, spinach, nutritional yeast, red

pepper flakes, salt, and pepper. Cook until the spinach is wilted.

11. Remove the skillet from the heat and stir in the tofu until combined well.

12. Taste and adjust seasoning. Spoon the tofu/spinach mixture into the baked crust and smooth out with a spoon.

13. Bake the quiche, uncovered, at 375F until the quiche is firm to the touch, about 33 to 37 minutes.

14. Remove from the oven and cool the quiche on a cooling rack for 15 to 20 minutes before slicing.

Nutritional Information Per Serving
- Calories 261
- Fat 16g
- Carbs 17.8g
- Protein 13.1g

Vegan Meatballs

Ingredients for 22 meatballs

For meatballs
- White onion – ½ cup, minced

- Garlic cloves – 3, minced
- Flax egg – 1 (1 tablespoon flaxseed meal and 2 ½ tablespoon water mixed together)
- Tempeh – 8 ounces
- Vegan parmesan cheese – 1/3 cup (raw cashews ¾ cup, nutritional yeast 3 tablespoons, sea salt ¾ teaspoon, and garlic powder ¼ teaspoon mix together in a food processor)
- Italian seasonings – 2 teaspoons
- Fresh parsley – ¼ cup
- Vegan bread crumbs – ½ cup
- Tomato sauce – 2 tablespoons
- Salt and pepper to taste
- Olive oil for sautéing

For coating
- Breadcrumbs - 1/3 cup
- Vegan parmesan cheese – 1/3 cup

Method
1. Preheat oven to 375F and in a small dish, prepare the flax egg.

2. In a large skillet, add ½ tablespoon olive oil and sauté onion and garlic over medium heat for 3 minutes, or until soft and translucent. Set aside.
3. Add tempeh to the food processor and pulse to break down. Then add sautéed onion, garlic (except olive oil) and remaining ingredients and mix. Make a dough.
4. Taste and adjust seasoning.
5. Scoop out about 1 tablespoon dough and roll into balls.
6. In a shallow bowl, mix parmesan cheese and remaining bread crumbs. Add the tempeh balls, one at a time and coat.
7. In the same skillet, add enough olive oil to form a thin layer on the bottom.
8. Then add the balls in two batches. Fry until all sides are browned, about 5 minutes total.
9. Add the browned meatballs to a baking sheet and bake in the oven until crisp, about 15 minutes.
10. Now prepare your favorite pasta.

11. Remove the meatballs once they are fairly firm to the touch and deep golden brown.
12. Top cooked pasta with meatballs and pour over the tomato sauce. Top with fresh parsley and vegan parmesan cheese.
13. Serve.

Nutritional Information Per Serving (1 meatball)
- Calories 66
- Fat 3.5g
- Carbs 6.1g
- Protein 3.2g

Veggie Burgers

Ingredients for 5 servings
- Cooked brown rice – 1 cup
- Raw walnuts – 1 cup
- Grape seed or avocado oil – ½ tablespoon plus more for cooking
- White onion – ¾ cup, finely diced

- Chili powder, smoked paprika and cumin powder – 1 tablespoon each
- Sea salt and black pepper – ½ teaspoon each, plus more for coating burgers
- Coconut sugar – 1 tablespoon
- Cooked black beans – 1 ½ cup, well rinsed, drained and patted dry
- Panko bread crumbs – 1/3 cup
- Vegan BBQ sauce – 3 to 4 tablespoons

Method

1. Add raw walnuts in a hot skillet and toast over medium heat until fragrant and golden brown, about 5 to 7 minutes, stirring frequently. Set aside.
2. Heat the same skillet over medium heat.
3. Add ½ tablespoon oil and onion. Season with salt and pepper and sauté until onion is soft, fragrant and translucent, about 3 to 4 minutes. Remove from heat and set aside.
4. In a food processor, add cooled walnuts, coconut sugar, smoked paprika, cumin, chili powder, salt and

pepper and blend until a fine meal is achieved. Set aside.

5. To a large bowl, add black beans and mash with a fork. Leave only a few beans whole.

6. Add spice-walnut mixture, sautéed onion, cooked rice, BBQ sauce, panko bread crumbs and mix with a wooden spoon until moldable dough forms, about 1 to 2 minutes. If too wet, add more breadcrumbs, if too dry, add 1 or 2 tablespoon BBQ sauce. Taste and adjust seasonings as needed.

7. Divide into 5 patties and set on baking sheet for grilling.

8. Heat the grill and brush the grill surface with oil.

9. Add the burgers to the grill and close the lid.

10. Cook until well browned on the underside, about 3 to 4 minutes, then flip gently.

11. Cook for 3 to 4 minutes on the other side.

12. Remove burgers from heat and let cool slightly.

13. Toast the buns and prepare your toppings.
14. Arrange and serve.

Nutritional Information Per Serving (1 burger without toppings or bun)
- Calories 392
- Fat 16.3g
- Carbs 52.1g
- Protein 13.6g

Baked Lentils with Sweet Potato

Ingredients for 4 servings
- Dry green lentils – 2 cups, rinsed and drained
- Sweet onion – 1, diced
- Garlic cloves – 3, minced
- Sweet apple – 1, peeled and diced
- Sweet potato – 1 medium, peeled and diced small
- Diced tomatoes – 1 (14-oz.) can
- Pure maple syrup – 2.5 tablespoons
- Blackstrap molasses – 2 tablespoons
- Regular mustard – 2 teaspoons

- Fine grain salt – ½ to 1 teaspoon
- Ground pepper to taste
- Apple cider vinegar – 1 to 2.5 tablespoons

Method

1. In a Dutch oven or a large oven-safe pot, add the lentils with 4 cups of water.
2. Bring the mixture to a boil, then lower the heat to low-medium and simmer, uncovered, until lentils are just tender and most of the water is absorbed, about 30 minutes. Stir often and add more water if needed.
3. Preheat the oven to 375F. Add the tomatoes (with juice), sweet potato, apple, garlic, onion, blackstrap molasses, maple syrup, mustard, salt and pepper to the pot with the lentils. Stir to combine. Add ½ of the apple cider vinegar.
4. Cover with a lid and bake at 375F for 20 to 25 minutes.
5. Remove from oven, uncover and stir.

6. Bake uncover until the sweet potato is tender, about 8 to 12 minutes more.
7. Stir the rest of the apple cider vinegar and season with salt and pepper.
8. Serve with a salad or toasted bread.

Nutritional Information Per Serving
- Calories 399
- Fat 1g
- Carbs 80.9g
- Protein 17.7g

Vegan Sandwich

Ingredients for 2 to 3 servings
Sandwich
- Chickpeas – 1 (15-ounce) can rinsed and drained
- Roasted unsalted sunflower seeds – ¼ cup
- Vegan mayo or tahini – 3 tablespoons
- Dijon or spicy mustard – ½ teaspoon
- Maple syrup – 1 tablespoon

- Chopped red onion – ¼ cup
- Fresh dill – 2 tablespoons, finely chopped
- Salt and pepper to taste
- Rustic bread – 4 pieces, lightly toasted
- Sliced onion, tomato, avocado, and lettuce for serving

Garlic Herb Sauce
- Hummus – ¼ cup
- Lemon juice – 1 tablespoon
- Dried dill – ¾ to 1 teaspoon
- Garlic – 2 cloves, minced
- Unsweetened almond milk to thin
- Sea salt to taste

Method
1. Prepare garlic herb sauce and set aside. To a mixing bowl, add the chickpeas and lightly mash with a fork.
2. Then add dill, red onion, maple syrup, mustard, mayo, sunflower seeds, salt and pepper and mix with a spoon.
3. Toast bread and prepare your toppings.
4. Arrange the sandwich and serve.

Nutritional Information Per Serving (without bread, sauce or toppings)

- Calories 311
- Fat 16g
- Carbs 26g
- Protein 11.5g

Vegan Pizza

Ingredients for 2 servings

Pizza

- Trader Joe's garlic-herb pizza crust – ½
- Green, red and orange bell pepper – ½ cup each, loosely chopped
- Red onion – 1/3 cup, chopped
- Button mushrooms - 1 cup, chopped
- Dried or fresh basil, garlic powder, and oregano – ½ teaspoon each
- Sea salt – ¼ teaspoon

Sauce

- Tomato sauce – 1 (15-ounce) can

- Oregano, garlic powder, dried or fresh basil, granulated sugar – ½ teaspoon each
- Sea salt to taste

Toppings
- Vegan parmesan cheese – ½ cup
- Red pepper flake and dried oregano

Method
1. Preheat the oven to 425F and place a rack in the center of the oven.
2. Heat 1 tablespoon olive oil in a large skillet over medium heat. Add the onion and peppers and season with herbs and salt. Stir and cook for 10 to 15 minutes, or until soft and slightly charred. Add the mushrooms in the last few minutes. Set aside.
3. Prepare the sauce: in a bowl, add tomato sauce, seasonings, and salt to taste. Set aside.
4. Onto a floured surface, roll out dough and transfer to a parchment-lined round baking sheet.

5. Top with tomato sauce, the sautéed veggies and a sprinkle of parmesan cheese.
6. Use the parchment lined baking sheet to slide the pizza directly onto the oven rack.
7. Bake until crisp and golden brown, about 17 to 20 minutes.
8. Serve with red pepper flake, dried oregano and parmesan cheese.

Nutritional Information Per Serving (1/2 pizza)
- Calories 395
- Fat 13g
- Carbs 59g
- Protein 15g

Chapter 4 Desserts

2-Layer No Bake Brownie Bars

Ingredients for 20 servings

Brownie Layer

- Raw walnuts – 1 cup
- Raw almonds – ½ cup
- Dates – 1 cups, pitted
- Non-dairy dark chocolate chips – ¼ cup
- Unsweetened cocoa powder – ½ cup plus 1 tablespoon
- Pinch of salt

Peanut Butter Layer

- Dates – ½ cup, pitted
- Raw almonds – ½ cup
- Roasted salted pecans – 1 cup
- Natural salted peanut butter – ½ cup

Method

1. To make the brown layer: in a food processor, pulse the dates until small bits remain. Remove from the processor and set aside in a bowl.
2. Add cocoa powder, chocolate chips, almonds and walnuts in the processor and pulse until well combined. Keep

the processor running and drop small bits of dates to form a dough. If the mixture is too dry, add a couple more pitted dates.

3. Press the dough into an 8 x 8 pan lined with parchment paper.
4. Press to make it flat and place in the freezer.
5. To make the peanut butter layer: in the food processor, press dates until small bits remain. Remove and set aside.
6. Then add peanuts and almonds and pulse until small bits remain. Add back in the dates and peanut butter and process until mixed.
7. Press on the top of the brownie layer until smooth.
8. Freeze for 15 to 20 minutes.
9. Then remove from pan and cut into 20 squares.
10. Serve.

Vegan Cheesecakes

Ingredients for 12 servings

Crust
- Pitted dates – 1 cup
- Raw almonds – 1 cup

Filling
- Raw cashews – 1 ½ cups, quick soaked
- Lemon juice – ¼ cup
- Coconut oil – 1/3 cup, melted
- Full-fat coconut milk – ½ cup plus 2 tablespoons
- Maple syrup – ½ cup

Flavor Add-Ins (optional)
- Salted natural peanut butter – 2 tablespoons
- Wild blueberries – ¼ cup
- Caramel sauce – 3 tablespoons

Method
1. In a food processor, add the dates and blend until small bits remain. Remove and set aside.
2. Now add the nuts and process into a meal. Add the dates back in and blend to make a loose dough. If too wet, add

37

more walnut or almond meal and if too dry, add a few dates.

3. Lightly grease a 12 slot muffin tin, then line the slots with parchment paper.

4. Scoop in 1 tablespoon amounts of crust and press with your fingers. Use the back of a spoon or a small glass to compact it and press it down. Set in the freezer to firm up.

5. In a blender, add all filling ingredients and mix until very smooth.

6. Taste and adjust seasonings as needed. Add the peanut butter and mix until combined. If flavoring with caramel or blueberry, wait and swirl on top of plain cheesecakes.

7. Split the filling evenly between the muffin tins. Release any air bubbles by tapping a few times.

8. Cover with a plastic wrap and freeze for 4 to 6 hours, or until hard.

9. Serve.

Nutritional Information Per Serving (1 cheesecake)

- Calories 324
- Fat 22g
- Carbs 29g
- Protein 6g

Vegan Chocolate Lava Cakes

Ingredients for 2 servings

- Unsweetened apple sauce – ¼ cup
- Unsweetened almond milk – ¼ cup + lemon juice or vinegar ½ teaspoon
- Cane sugar – 2.5 tablespoons
- Melted coconut oil – 1 tablespoon
- Vanilla extract – ¼ teaspoon
- Baking powder – ¼ teaspoon
- Pinch sea salt
- Unsweetened cocoa powder – 2 tablespoons
- Unbleached all-purpose flour – ¼ cup plus ½ tablespoon
- Semisweet chocolate chips – 2 tablespoons, melted
- Vegan dark chocolate – 2 squares plus coconut whipped cream for topping

Method

1. Preheat the oven to 375F.

2. Use dairy-free butter to grease two standard size muffin tins, then coat with cocoa powder. Shake out excess.

3. In a small bowl, add the vinegar and almond milk and mix. Set aside for a few minutes to activate.

4. Add the applesauce, vanilla, oil and sugar and beat until foamy. Then add the flour, cocoa powder, baking powder, and salt. Mix so no lumps remain.

5. Add the melted semisweet chocolate and mix.

6. Divide the batter evenly between two muffin tins.

7. Break up one square of the dark chocolate and press it down into the middle of the cakes. Cover with batter.

8. Bake until the top is no longer wet and the edges have pulled away slightly, about 15 to 20 minutes.

9. Let rest in the pan for 5 minutes before removing. Then gently transfer to serving plates.

10. Top each cake with the remaining square of dark chocolate and serve with coconut whipped cream.

Nutritional Information Per Serving (1 cake)
- Calories 353
- Fat 16g
- Carbs 51g
- Protein 4g

Vegan Cookies

Ingredients for 2 dozen
Ingredients
- Dates – 1 cup (soaked in warm water for 10 minutes, then drained)
- Ripe banana – 1 medium
- Natural salted almond or peanut butter – 2 tablespoons
- Almond meal – ¾ cup
- Gluten free rolled oats – ¾ cup
- Optional add-ins: nuts, dried fruits, dairy-free chocolate chips

Method

1. In a food processor, pulse the dates until small bits remain.
2. Add almond butter and banana and mix until combined.
3. Add the rolled oats and almond meal and pulse until a loose dough is formed.
4. Scrape the dough into a mixing bowl. If it feels too wet, add a few tablespoons of almond meal and stir.
5. Add ¼ cup of add-ins of your choice, such as nuts, raisins or dark chocolate chips. Then chill the dough for 10 minutes.
6. Preheat the oven to 350F.
7. Scoop out about 1 tablespoon of cookie dough and make loose discs. Arrange them on a parchment lined baking sheet.
8. Bake until golden brown and somewhat firm to the touch, about 15 to 18 minutes.
9. Remove from the oven and cool for a few minutes.

10.Serve.

Nutritional Information Per Serving (1 cookie)
- Calories 75
- Fat 3.2g
- Carbs 11.4g
- Protein 1.6g

Vegan Banana Cream Pie

Ingredients for 8 servings

Crust
- Walnuts – 1 heaping cup
- Pitted dates – 1 heaping cup (soaked in warm water for 10 minutes, then drained)

Filling
- Cashews – 1.2 cups (soaked overnight and drained)
- Coconut oil – 3.5 tablespoons, melted

- Maple syrup – ¼ cup
- Just ripe banana – 1 medium, mashed
- Full-fat coconut milk – 1/3 cup
- Pure vanilla extract – ½ teaspoon
- Sea salt - ¼ teaspoon
- Lemon juice – 2 to 3 tablespoons

Method

1. In the food processor, process dates until small bits remain. Remove and set aside.
2. Process walnuts until a meal consistency is achieved.
3. Add back in dates and a pinch of salt and mix to combine.
4. It the mixture is too wet, add a little walnut or almond meal, if the mixture is too dry, add another date or two.
5. Press into an 8 x 8 baking dish lined with parchment. Press until flat, going up the sides (about ½ inch). Place in the freezer to set.
6. In a blender, add all the filling ingredients and blend for 1 to 2 minutes, or until smooth and creamy.

7. Taste and adjust seasoning as needed and add a spoonful of peanut butter.
8. Then pour into crust and smooth with a spoon.
9. Cover and freeze for 4 to 6 hours, or until set.
10. To serve, let thaw for 5 minutes.
11. Then top slices with crushed peanuts and coconut whipped cream.

Nutritional Information Per Serving (1 slice without toppings)
- Calories 391
- Fat 27g
- Carbs 35g
- Protein 8g

Conclusion

As you can see this vegan cookbook contains delicious and simple recipes that will help you lose weight and achieve all of your health goals.

Part 2

Introduction

Veggie lover diets differ extensively relying upon the level of dietary confinements. As indicated by the strictest definition, a veggie lover diet comprises basically of grains, organic products, vegetables, vegetables, and nuts; creature sustenance, including milk, dairy items, and eggs by and large are avoided. A few less prohibitive veggie lover eating methodologies may incorporate eggs and dairy items. Some vegan weight control plans might be gathered as takes after:

Macrobiotic

Vegetables, natural products, vegetables, and kelp are incorporated into the eating routine, while entire grains, particularly cocoa rice, are likewise stressed. Privately developed organic products are prescribed. Creature nourishments constrained to white meat or white-meat fish might be incorporated into the eating regimen more than once every week.

Semi-vegan

Meat periodically is incorporated into the eating regimen. Some individuals who take after such an eating regimen may not eat red meat but rather may eat fish and maybe chicken.

Lacto-vegetarian

Eggs, drain, and drain items (lacto = dairy; ovo = eggs) are incorporated, yet no meat is expended.

Lactovegetarian

Milk and drain items are incorporated into the eating regimen, however no eggs or meat are expended.

Veggie lover

All creature items, including eggs, drain, and drain items, are rejected from the eating regimen. A few vegetarians don't utilize nectar and may cease from utilizing creature items, for example, cowhide or fleece. They likewise may stay away from nourishments that are handled or not naturally developed.

1. Delicious Cilantro Pistou

Ingredients

- 4 cups cilantro leaves
- 6 cloves garlic, peeled
- ½ cup olive oil
- ½ tsp. salt, optional
- ? tsp. freshly ground black pepper

Method

1. Mix cilantro and garlic in food processor till finely sliced.
2. Now blend in oil. Flavor with salt and pepper.

2. Healthy Quinoa Tabbouleh

Ingredients

- 1½ cups of quinoa
- 1¾ tsp. of fine sea salt, divided
- olive oil
- ¾ cup of lemon juice
- 2 cloves of garlic, minced
- ½ tsp. of freshly ground black pepper
- 2 cups of diced tomatoes or quartered cherry tomatoes
- 1½ cups of parsley, chopped
- 3 unpeeled Persian cucumbers, diced
- 4 green onions, thinly sliced
- ½ cup of fresh mint leaves, chopped

Method

1. Rinse quinoa in water and drain.
2. Heat skillet and add quinoa, and toast 10 minutes, or till moisture vanishes and quinoa is fragrant and golden, stir continually with (flat-tipped) spoon or rice paddle.

3. Boil 21/2 cups water in saucepan. Now add 1/4 tsp. salt, then quinoa. Reduce heat to medium-low, cover pan, and simmer for approx. 20 minutes, or till quinoa is delicate. Fluff quinoa with a fork, and put into bowl to cool.

4. Mix together oil, garlic, pepper, lemon juice and remaining 1 1/2 tsp. salt in bowl.

5. Mix tomatoes, parsley, cucumbers, green onions, and mint into cooled quinoa. Put dressing over top. Serve till salad is cold.

3. Delicious Spinach, Peppers, and Cherry

Ingredients

- 2 ½ cups of penne rigate pasta
- 1 Tbs. of olive oil
- 2 cloves of garlic, minced (2 tsp.)
- 1 12-oz. of jar roasted red peppers, rinsed, drained, patted dry, and sliced
- 10 oz. of cherry tomatoes, halved (2 cups)

- 4 cups of packed baby spinach leaves (8 oz.)
- ¼ cup of hacked kalamata olives
- 1 Tbs. of chopped fresh oregano
- 1 ½ tsp. of grated lemon zest
- ¼ tsp. of ground black pepper

Method

1. Heat oil in large skillet over medium heat. Add garlic, and cook 1 for minute, stir frequently, or till lightly browned.
2. Set heat to high. Now add roasted peppers, and cook 3 - 4 minutes, or till lightly browned, stir sometimes.
3. Now add tomatoes, fresh spinach, olives, oregano, lemon zest, and pepper. Cook 4 - 6 minutes, or till tomatoes soften and spinach wilts, stir regularly. Combine pasta and (pasta-cooking) water; cover, and cook approx. 3 minutes more, or till heated.

4. Tasty Cauliflower Shawarma

Ingredients

- 1 tsp of cumin powder
- 1 tsp of coriander powder
- 1/2 tsp of paprika
- 1/4 tsp of ground black pepper
- 1/4 tsp of ground cinnamon
- 1/4 tsp of ground cardamom
- 1/8 tsp of ground cloves
- 1 tsp of garlic powder
- 1 small head of cauliflower, sliced into florets
- 1/4 cup of water
- 1/4 - 1/2 tsp of salt
- 2 tsp of oil
- 1/3 - 1/2 tsp of cayenne
- 1/2 tsp of garlic granules or 1 tsp garlic paste

Method

1. Mix all the spices and Prep the rest of the ingredients and tahini dressing.
2. In a skillet, now add cauliflower florets, water and salt and cover and cook over

medium heat for 12 - 14 minutes or till al dente.

3. In 2 tsp oil, combine in 2 - 3 tsp of the spice blend, garlic and cayenne. Put the oil on the cauliflower. Cook for 2 minutes or more till the spices start to smell roasted. Stir. Adjust salt and heat.

4. Heat the pita, and add warm cauliflower to the pitas, add tomatoes, cucumber, greens. Sprinkle tahini sauce. Drizzle cilantro or parsley. Serve.

5. Delicious Jackfruit Gyros

Ingredients

- 1 Tbs. of vegan margarine
- 1 onion, halved and thinly sliced
- 1 20-oz. of can young jackfruit in brine, rinsed, drained, and shreds
- ¾ cup of (low-sodium) vegetable broth
- 4 Tbs. of lemon juice, divided
- 2 tsp. of dried oregano
- 1 tsp. of (low-sodium) soy sauce
- ¾ tsp. of ground coriander

Method

1. Heat margarine in skillet till sizzling. Add onion, and sauté 3 - 4 minutes, or till softened. Now add jackfruit, and cook 20 minutes, or till browned and caramelized.

2. Add broth, 2 Tbs. of lemon juice, oregano, soy sauce, and coriander, and flavor with salt and pepper. Simmer 10 - 15 minutes.

3. Stir in rest 2 Tbs. of lemon juice.

6. Tasty Grape Leaves Casserole

Ingredients

- 1 large onion, finely diced
- 1 cup brown rice
- 2 cups low-Na(Sodium) tomato juice or vegetable juice
- 1 cup of sliced unsalted, hulled pistachios

- 1 cup of sliced fresh parsley
- 1 cup of sliced fresh mint
- 1 cup of raisins or dried currants
- ¼ cup of lemon juice
- 1 lemon, sliced, for garnish

Method

1. Dip grape leaves in boiling water 2 minutes. Drain, and set aside.
2. Heat oil in saucepan and add onion, and sauté 7 - 10 minutes, or till brown. Now add rice and 21/2 cups water, and boil. Cover and reduce heat to medium-low, then cook 30 - 40. Take away from heat, and stir in tomato juice, pistachios, parsley, mint, raisins, and lemon juice. Flavor with salt and pepper.
3. Heat oven to 350°F. Brush baking dish with olive oil and Pat grape leaves dry. Line bottom and sides of baking dish with grape leaves and spread half of rice mixture over grape leaves. Top rice with more grape leaves, then top with rest of rice mixture. Cover casserole

with remaining grape leaves, and seal by folding over grape leaving edges. Brush top with olive oil. Bake 30 - 40 minutes, or till grape leaves on top darken and casserole looks dry.

7. Healthy Spinach Artichoke Dip

Ingredients

- ½ white onion
- 2 cloves of garlic
- ½ cup of vegan cream cheese
- ½ cup of vegan sour cream
- ¾ cup of vegan mozzarella cheese shreds
- 1 cup of marinated artichoke hearts, chopped
- 2 cups of frozen spinach, thawed and drained
- Bread crumbs or panko

Method

1. Slice onion and garlic, and sauté in olive oil on low heat till translucent.

2. In a bowl, mix the onions and garlic with the cream cheese, sour cream, mozzarella shreds, chopped artichoke hearts, and spinach.
3. Now add freshly cracked pepper and a pinch of salt.
4. Put into oven safe dish and drizzle with breadcrumbs.
5. Bake at 375 for approx. 30 minutes.

8. Middle Eastern Red Lentil Soup

Ingredients

- 1 onion, sliced
- 3 tsp. olive oil
- 3 cloves garlic, sliced
- 1½ tsp cumin
- 1½ tsp ground coriander
- pinch of ground cayenne
- 1¾ cup split red lentils
- bunch of fresh celery leaves, sliced
- 1 carrot, sliced
- 2 quart vegetable stock

- salt and pepper to taste
- juice of one lemon

Method

1. In a pot, soften onion in oil over moderate heat for 2-3 minutes.
2. Add garlic, cumin, coriander, and cayenne. Stir and mix the spices for 1-2 minute.
3. Stirring in the lentils, celery leaves, and carrot. Cover with stock, and boil, stir sometimes
4. Decrease heat and simmer 35-45 minutes or till lentils are soft.
5. Add salt and pepper to taste.
6. Puree soup in a blendert.
7. Stir in lemon juice.
8. Garnish with vegan sour cream, minced carrots.

9. Delicious Cilantro Hummus

Ingredients

- 1 can of garbanzo beans
- 5 cloves of garlic
- 1 dried red chili pepper
- 1 tsp of black pepper
- 1 tsp of tahini sauce
- 1/2 tsp of salt
- 1 Tsp. of lime juice
- 1/2 tsp of rock salt
- 1 cup of chopped cilantro
- 3 tsps of olive oil
- 1 tsp of cayenne pepper

Method

1. Heat 2 tsp olive oil.
2. Now add the red chili pepper and the garlic cloves.
3. Heat the garlic for 5 minutes stir sometimes.
4. Now add in the garbanzo beans, spices and mix well for 2 minutes.
5. Blend with cilantro leaves and a little water.
6. Drizzle the remaining olive oil and cayenne pepper before serving.

10. Delicious Bean Burgers

Ingredients

- 2 cans of kidney beans, drained and rinsed
- 1 - 2 medium to large cloves garlic
- 2 1/2 tsp. of tomato paste
- 1 1/2 tsp. of red wine
- 1 tsp of Dijon mustard
- 3/4 cup green onions, sliced
- 1/4 cup fresh parsley, roughly chopped
- 2 tsp. of fresh oregano, chopped
- 1/2 tsp of sea salt
- freshly ground black pepper to taste
- 1 1/4 cups of rolled oats
- 1/3 – 1/2 cup of kalamata olives, roughly chopped
- 1/4 cup of diced red bell pepper

Method

1. Mix the kidney beans, garlic, tomato paste, vinegar, and mustard in a food processor, Mix till pureed. Now add the

green onions, parsley, oregano, salt, and pepper to taste. Add the oats and pulse to begin to incorporate.

2. Pour the mixture into a bowl and stir in the olives and red pepper. Refrigerate the mixture for 30 - 45 minutes, then shape into patties with your hands. To cook, wipe a smidgen of oil over a skillet on medium-high heat. Cook the patties for 6 to 8 minutes per side.

11. Mediterranean Stir Fry

Ingredients

- 1/4 pumpkin, thinly cut
- 1 bunch of asparagus, cut
- 2 zucchini , thinly cut
- 1 eggplant , salted, thinly slice
- 1 bunch of bok choy
- 400 gram of red kidney beans, cooked
- 1 cup of brown rice
- 3 cups of water
- Olive oil

- Black pepper
- Rosemary
- Basil

Method

1. Boil 3 cups of water, then add brown rice, heat till cooked.
2. Mix olive oil with pepper, rosemary, and basil in heated wok.
3. Now add pumpkin, asparagus and zucchini, stir-fry.
4. Combine eggplant, mix till soft.
5. Add bok choy and kidney beans, stir.
6. Serve with rice.

12. Homemade Delicious Hummus

Ingredients

- 200 gram of chickpeas
- 3 tsp. of olive oil
- juice of a lemon
- 2 bay of leaves
- 1 clove of garlic

- 1 tsp of tahini sauce or 1 tsp. sesame oil
- salt and black ground pepper, to taste

Method

1. Keep the chickpeas in water for 24 hours before cooking.
2. Boil the chickpeas for around two hours with by, then remove the bay leaf and keep a glass of the liquid.
3. Blend the chickpeas with the garlic, a little bit of salt, the liquid, the olive oil, the tahini/sesame and some black pepper.
4. To get the flavor and texture you like, try different amounts of ingredients, depending on your taste.

13. Amazing Vegan Recipe

Ingredients

- 1 large eggplant
- 2-4 cloves fresh garlic
- 1-2 tsp. olive oil

- 1 freshly squeezed lemon
- 1 tsp paprika or ground red pepper
- 1-2 tsp. tahini
- 1/2 cup chopped fresh parsley
- sea salt to taste

Method

1. Heat oven to 350F degrees. Wrapping the eggplant in tin foil, and set it onto the upper rack.
2. Put rest of ingredients into a blender, and select the (chop) setting to mix everything and slice the garlic.
3. Bake eggplant for 30-45 minutes. Take it out
4. Cut top and then cut it in half.
5. Dice it up, and then put cubes into blender with other ingredients. Select (chop) and blend mixture till thoroughly mixed.
6. Transfer into a dish and set aside for approx. 10 minutes. Serve with toasted Syrian flat bread.

14. Tasty Puckery Pomegranate Seitan

Ingredients

- 2 tsp. of oil
- 1 lb. of seitan, cut into chops
- 1 onion, cut
- 2 cloves garlic, shredded
- salt and pepper to taste
- 4 tsp. of pomegranate molasses
- 2/3 cup of vegetable stock, plus more for deglazing the pan if necessary
- 1/4 cup of walnuts
- dash of sugar

Method

1. Fry the seitan for 5 minutes or till it starts browning and remove seitan from.
2. In the same pan, saute onions, garlic, salt, and pepper till the onion softens. Combine pomegranate molasses, stock,

walnuts, and sugar, and bring to a simmer.

3. Put seitan back to the pan and coat with sauce.

15. Delicious Spring Hummus

Ingredients

- 1/4 cup of lemon juice
- 1 tsp. of tahini
- 1/2 tsp. of chopped garlic (more or less to taste)
- 1 tsp of sea salt
- 1/2 tsp of cumin
- 1/4 tsp of cayenne pepper

Method

1. Put all ingredients in a food processor, and process till smooth. Serve it warm or chilled.

16.Tahini Sauce

Ingredients

- 1/2 cup sesame paste
- 1 tsp garlic salt
- 1 tsp lemon salt
- 1 tsp vinegar
- 1/2 cup Italian dressing

Method

1. Mix all ingredients in a food processor, and blend till smooth.
2. Add water if mixture is too thick.
3. Serve with falafels in a sandwich

17. Delicious Falafels

Ingredients

- 16 ounce or 2 cans of cooked chickpeas
- 1/2 cup of whole wheat flour
- 1 clove of garlic
- 1 tsp. of salt

- 3 dashes of Tabasco or chili sauce
- cooking oil

Instructions

1. Grind all falafel ingredients in a food processor till mixture holds together when formed in balls.
2. Then add more flour if watery. Deep roast falafel balls in oil.

18. Delicious Tabouli

Ingredients

- 1 tomato, seeded and diced
- 1 1/2 cup fresh parsley, minced
- 2 tsp. green onion, chopped
- 2 tsp. fresh mint, minced
- 3 tsp fresh lemon juice
- 3 tsp olive oil
- pinch of sea salt, to taste

Instructions

1. In a bowl mix all ingredients well. Keep Tabouli for 3 days in a sealed container in the refrigerator.

19. Best Hummus

Ingredients

- 1 1/2 cup garbanzo beans, cooked and drained
- 1 tsp. tahini
- 1 tsp olive oil
- 3 tsp. lemon juice
- 1/4 cup water
- 1 large clove fresh garlic, minced
- 1/2 tsp ground cumin
- pinch of red chili pepper powder
- 1/2 cup fresh cilantro, chopped

Method

1. In blender, puree all ingredients except cilantro. Put puree into a bowl. Now

stir in cilantro leaves. Serve with pita
bread like carrots and celery sticks.

20. Healthy Baba Ganouj

Ingredients

- 4 eggplants
- 2 lemons, juice
- 6 cloves of garlic
- 1 cup of chopped parsley
- 1/2 cup of scallions, finely sliced
- 1 cup of tahini
- 2 tsps of of salt
- black pepper
- olive oil

Method

1. Heat oven to 400F degrees. Wash and
   remove stem eggplants. Prick eggplants
   all around, and put directly on an oven
   rack.

2. Roast eggplants for approx. 45-50 minutes till they become wrinkled and very soft. Remove it from oven and let it cool. Scoop the insides of eggplant put into a bowl, and mash.
3. Add all rest of ingredients except olive oil and mix. Let it chill, drizzle with olive oil, and serve.

21. Delicious Mediterranean Stew

Ingredients

- 1 medium eggplant, chopped
- 2 medium zucchini, chopped
- 1 green pepper chopped
- 1 onion chopped
- 3 tomatoes chopped
- 30 ounce garbanzo beans, pre-cooked, rinsed and drained
- 9 ounce frozen artichokes, quartered
- 1 tsp. oregano
- salt, pepper, and red pepper flakes to taste

Method

1. Combine all ingredients in cooking pot and cook till heated through and zucchini is tender. Serve with rice, noodles, or couscous.

22. Tasty Tabbouleh

Ingredients

- 1 cup of bulgur wheat
- 1 cup of hot (not boiling) water
- 1 lemon, juice
- 1/2 cup of olive oil
- 1 cup of parsley finely chopped
- 1/2 cup of green onion finely chopped
- 2 tsp of minced garlic
- 4 roma tomatoes diced
- 1 cucumber diced
- 1/4-1/2 tsp of sea salt and freshly ground pepper to taste

Method

1. Mix bulgur, water, and lemon juice in a bowl. Set aside it for 30 minutes, then fluff it with a fork to isolate the grains. Add rest of ingredients and combine.
2. Flavors will be intensified after a while. Cover and refrigerate at least 2 hours before serving

23. Mediterranean Delicious Pasta Salad

Ingredients

Salad:
- ½ lb. of short pasta
- 1 (14 oz) can quartered artichoke hearts in brine, coarsely chopped
- ½ small white onion, cut
- ½ cup of sliced flat parsley leaves
- ¼ cup of Kalamata olives, pitted and sliced

- ¼ cup of sundried tomatoes in extra-virgin olive oil with Italian herbs, sliced small
- ¼ cup of toasted pine nuts
- ¼ cup of Grated Parmesan Topping

Dressing:

- 6 tsp. of sundried tomato oil
- 4 tsp. of balsamic vinegar
- 1½ tsp. of maple syrup or agave (see Note)
- 1 small clove garlic, grated
- ½ tsp of Dijon mustard
- ½ tsp of crushed red pepper flakes (more or less to taste)
- ½ tsp of salt
- black pepper to taste

Method

1. Cook the pasta. Now drain and set aside to cool.
2. Mix all ingredients for the dressing in a bowl.
3. When the pasta is cool, rinse under cold water; drain it well, and put it into

the bowl. Now add the artichoke hearts, onion, parsley, olives, sundried tomatoes, pine nuts, and Parmesan Topping, and gently combine.
4. Serve.

24. Delicious Sicilian Caponata

Ingredients

- 4 tbsp of olive oil
- 2 eggplants, chopped
- 1 onion, diced
- 1 green bell pepper, deseeded and diced
- 6-8 plum tomatoes, chopped
- 1 carrot, chopped
- 2 tsp of fresh basil or 1 tsp dried basil
- 1/2 cup of green olives, chopped
- 1-2 tbsp of capers
- 1 tsp of dried oregano
- 1 tsp of salt
- 1 tsp of sugar
- raisins

Method

1. In a large pan, heat the olive oil. Add everything to the pot and simmer on medium heat for about an hour. Serve!

25. Delicious Spanish Croquetas

Ingredients

- 10-12 ripe tomatoes, skinned
- 1/2 cucumber, skinned
- 1/2 red bell pepper
- 2 cloves of garlic
- 1/3 baguette bread
- Salt to taste
- 1/2 cup olive oil

Method

1. Boil water and add the whole tomatoes for 5 minutes and remove. The skin will come right off. In a blender, add all of the ingredients and blend till smooth.

2. After blend, run all of the gazpacho through a strainer. Strain all of the soup into the bowl.

26. Delicious Sicilian broccoli

Ingredients

- 3 tbsp olive oil
- 1 onion, sliced
- 3 cups broccoli, florets
- 1/3 cup black olives, sliced (optional)
- 1 cup water
- 1 cup red wine
- 1 tsp salt

Method

1. In a pot, heat the olive oil and add the sliced onion. Cook till the onions are soft and add the broccoli. Then stir for a few minutes and add one cup of water and some salt.

2. Cook, stir the broccoli till the water evaporates and now add the wine. Then stir for another 15 minutes

27. Amazing Risi e Bisi

Ingredients

- 1 onion, chopped
- 4 tbsp of margarine
- 1 tbsp of parsley
- Salt to taste
- 1/2 tsp of pepper
- 2 cups of fresh or frozen peas
- 1/2 cup of white wine
- 2 cups of short grain rice, dry
- 7 cups of vegetable broth, hot

Method

1. In a pan, melt 3 tbsp margarine and add the chopped onion. Fry for around 10 minutes or till the onions are translucent.

2. Now add the salt, pepper, spices, and peas and fry for another 5 minutes. Transfer the wine into the pan and stir for around 3 minutes. Now add the dry rice and stir till it has soaked up all of the liquid.
3. Put in the broth, cup by cup, while constantly stirring for 20-25 minutes or till the rice is cooked. Now put 1 tbsp of margarine on removing the risotto from heat and serve.

28. Tasty Catalan Escalivada

Ingredients

- Eggplants
- Red bell peppers
- Sweet onions
- Tomatoes
- Olive Oil
- Salt

Method

1. Heat the oven to 500 F (260 C). Drizzle the whole vegetables with olive oil and put them on an oven tray.
2. Put in oven for 35-40 minutes, turning twice. The vegetables must be charred when you take out. Let it cool and put off the skin and seeds of all the vegetables. Cut into strips, drizzle with olive oil and salt.

29. Amazing Catalan Trinxat

Ingredients

- 2 large potatoes, peeled and chopped
- 1/2 head of green cabbage, chopped
- 2 cloves garlic, minced
- 3 tbsp olive oil
- tsp salt

Method

1. In a pot, boil the sliced potatoes and cabbage for 30 minutes. In a pan, fry

the crushed garlic in 1 tbsp olive oil till lightly browned.

2. Strain the potatoes and cabbage in a colander and put them in a bowl. Mash the potatoes and cabbage with the garlic till smooth. Form the patties of the mashed potatoes and fry in a pan in olive oil till browned on both sides.

30. Delicious Turkish Miroloto

Ingredients

- 4 cups of corn flour
- 1/2 cup of margarine or 1/4 cup of oil
- 1 tsp of salt
- 3 tsp of baking powder
- 2 cups of chopped greens
- 1 onion, chopped
- 2 1/2 - 3 cups of water
- 2 tbsp of olive oil

Method

1. In a bowl, mix the flour, baking powder, and salt. Mix the margarine or oil. Put the water, onion, and greens and mix till a thick dough has formed.
2. In a pan or skillet, heat the 2 tbsp of olive oil. Press the dough and cover. Heat for 30 minutes. Take away cover and cook for 10 minutes more.

31. Turkish Mantarli

- 3 tbsp of olive oil
- 10-12 mushrooms, sliced
- 1 bundle of asparagus, sliced
- 1 tsp. of salt
- 1/2 tsp. of pepper
- 3 tsp. of lemon zest or lemon juice
- 2 cups of cooked rice

Method

1. In a pan, heat the 3 tbsp. of olive oil on medium-high heat. Add the sliced mushrooms, asparagus, salt, pepper, and lemon zest and fry for 10 minutes.

2. Add the cooked rice and mix for another 3 minutes. Serve hot or cold.

32. Mediterranean Tasty Quinoa

Ingredients

- 1 cup of quinoa
- 2 tsp. of oil, divided
- 4 cloves of garlic, minced, divided
- 8 ounces button mushrooms, thinly cut
- 2 red pepper, thinly cut
- 1/4-1/2 cup feta, diced
- handful fresh basil
- 1 tsp. of lemon juice
- Salt and pepper to taste

Method

1. In a pot add 1 tsp. oil and cook half of the garlic over medium heat till aromatic. Then add quinoa and cook till lightly browned. Add 1 1/2 cups of water, boil and decrease heat and

simmer, covered for 20 minutes or till cooked through.

2. In a pan heat rest of oil over medium heat and add peppers. Heat till lightly cooked through and add garlic. Cook till aromatic. Take away from pan. To the same pan, now add mushrooms and cook till lightly browned on both sides.

3. When quinoa is cooked through mix quinoa with mushrooms, peppers, garlic, basil, lemon juice and feta. Toss till mixed.

33. Tasty Eggplant and Feta Dip

Ingredients

- 1 medium eggplant
- Eggplant
- 2 tsp. of lemon juice
- 1/4 cup of extra-virgin olive oil
- 1/2 cup of crumbled feta cheese
- 1/2 cup of finely sliced red onion
- 1 red bell pepper, finely sliced

- 1 chili pepper, such as jalapeño, seeded and crushed
- 2 tsp. of sliced fresh basil
- 1 tsp. of finely sliced flat-leaf parsley
- 1/4 tsp of cayenne pepper, or to taste
- 1/4 tsp of salt

Method

1. Preheat broiler.
2. Now line a baking pan with foil. Put eggplant in the pan and make a few holes all over it to vent steam. Broil the eggplant, turn with tongs after approx. 5 minutes, till the skin is overcooked. Put into a cutting board till cool enough to handle.
3. Put lemon juice in a bowl. Cut the eggplant in half and put the flesh into the bowl, tossing with the lemon juice. Put oil and stir with a fork till the oil is absorbed. Now stir in feta, onion, bell pepper, chili pepper, basil, parsley, cayenne and salt. Add sugar if needed.

34. Healthy Lemon Chickpeas with Spinach

Ingredients

- 1 tbsp of coconut oil
- 1 small onion, sliced
- 2 cloves garlic, minced
- 2 cups of cooked chickpeas
- 2 tbsp of fresh dill, finely chopped
- 3 tbsp of fresh lemon juice
- salt and pepper, to taste
- 1 bunch of spinach, stemmed and sliced

Method

1. In a skillet over medium heat, add oil. When hot, add onion and fry till softened, about 5 minutes. Put in garlic and fry for 1 minute more.
2. Put in chickpeas and dill and cook for 2 minutes, till heated through. Deglaze

with the lemon juice and flavor to taste. Stir in half of the spinach till it wilts and then add the rest of spinach. Cover, cook till wilted, 1-2 minutes tops. Serve with rice or quinoa.

35. Tasty Chickpea Salad with Lemon

Ingredients

- 1/2 pint of cherry tomatoes, sliced in half
- 6 oz. mozzarella cheese, cubed
- 1/2 red pepper, sliced
- 1/2 cucumber, sliced
- 2-16 oz cans of chickpeas, rinsed
- 2 celery stalks, leaves removed and sliced
- 1/2 sweet onion, sliced
- 3 garlic cloves, minced
- 3 Tbsp. of extra virgin olive oil
- 1 Tbsp. of red wine vinegar
- 1/2 lemon, juiced
- 1/2 tsp. of cumin

- 1/2 tsp. of paprika
- 1/2 tsp. of basil
- Fresh parsley, chopped
- Pepper to taste

Method

1. In a mixing bowl mix tomatoes, cucumber, chickpeas, mozzarella cheese, red pepper, celery and sweet onion.
2. In a salad dressing container or bowl mix garlic, extra virgin olive oil, red wine vinegar, lemon juice, cumin, paprika and basil.
3. Put dressing over the salad and mix.
4. in salt and pepper to taste.

About the Author

Fred Ivey is author of several cookbooks on Vegan diet. He has written research papers on the topic and currently lives in California.

CPSIA information can be obtained
at www.ICGtesting.com
Printed in the USA
BVHW041429210120
570067BV00010B/392

9 781989 682913